I0839432

GET

FIT

(THE ULTIMATE GUIDE TO HEALTHY LIVING)

LATEEFAH RAJI

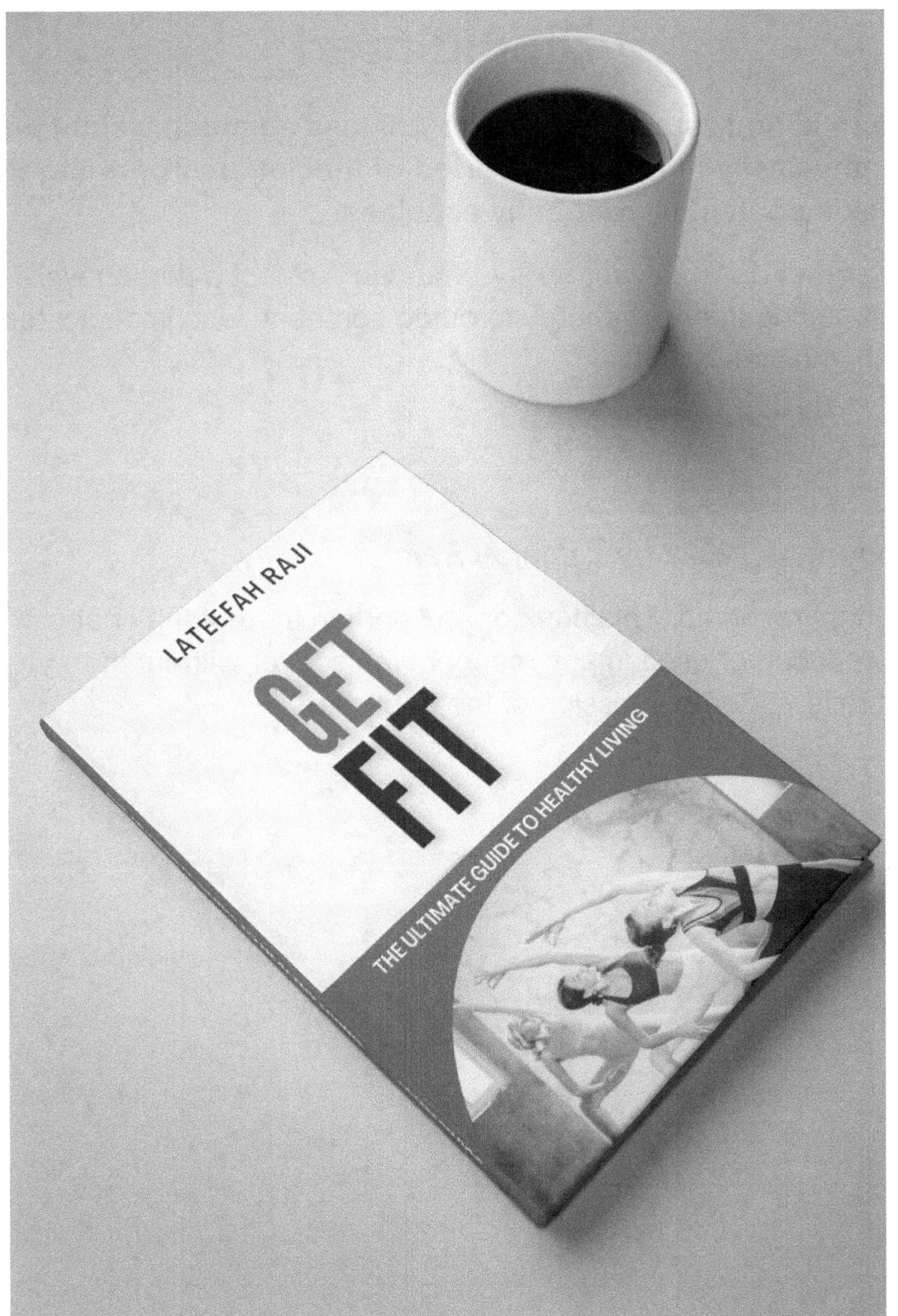

LATEEFAH RAJI
GET FIT
THE ULTIMATE GUIDE TO HEALTHY LIVING

Disclaimer!

There is no assurance that you will lose so much weight and be physically fit in a short period of time of incorporating this book's content in your daily activities.

It narrows down to your ability. You can't expect a person who isn't putting the right energy to outdo someone who is dedicated to the hustle!

Table of Contents

Introduction

What Does It Mean To Be Physically Fit?

Many of us have erroneous ideas about what being physically fit entails. For instance, some individuals believe that to be deemed fit, they must meet particular weight requirements, complete a marathon, or be able to bench press twice their body weight. Good for you if you fit any of these characteristics. However, you might not be as physically fit as you should be.

The fact is that physical fitness encompasses far more than simply your weight or how well you perform in one particular sport.

A useful definition of physical fitness is as follow:

- **It is a general condition of health and wellbeing that encompasses the capacity to carry out daily tasks and leisure activities with efficiency and the ability to fend against illness**.

It is incorrect to think that possessing a specific weight or having large muscles equates to being fit under these criteria. *Fitness is more about having the physical capacity to handle daily obligations.*

Now that's a little bit closer to the goal we ought to be aiming towards. *Being the fittest rather than just being sufficiently fit.*

So, the question is: What can you do to achieve the highest quality of life or to be the fittest version of yourself?

To answer that question, we'll examine the five components of physical fitness.

Components Of Physical Fitness

According to the criteria provided by the *Department of Health and Human Services*, improving physical fitness requires attention to five (5) crucial areas.

1. Muscular Endurance

The length of time your muscles can hold a position or perform an action repeatedly before becoming fatigued is known as muscular endurance.

How many repetitions of a specific weight you can perform in sets at the gym, as well as how many pull-ups and push-ups you can complete in a single session, are a few ways to measure your physical endurance.

Muscular endurance is useful for everyday chores like carrying groceries, mowing the lawn, or cradling a kid, even though we tend to think of exercise in terms of physical activity.

2. Muscular Power

Muscular strength is the capacity of a muscle to produce force during an activity, such as your maximum deadlift or bench press, your maximum resistance setting on a machine, or your capacity to pick something up off the ground.

Due to the way we live in the contemporary world, many of us have strength imbalances. For instance, despite having relatively weak glutes or hamstrings from working at a desk all day, you could be able to bench press heavy weight.

3. Structure Of The Body

It matters less how much you weigh than what percentage of bone, muscle, and fat is in your body. Even BMI measures which don't consider athletic builds might be misleading when used in isolation.

While some individuals who appear overweight may have a healthy body fat composition, others who appear fit may have a larger amount of body fat. Between 8 to 35 percent is the suggested range for women who have most body fat, and between 5 and 29 percent for males.

So how can you determine your level of body fat? Doctors and nutritionists may evaluate your body fat for you, and also personal trainers and fitness clubs have equipment like tape measures, calipers, and specialist scales.

4. Flexibility

All the muscular or cardiovascular endurance in the world wouldn't assist you if you weren't flexible.

The flexibility of a person is determined by the range of motion around each joint. Although you don't need to be a gymnast or yogi, keeping your muscles and bones flexible with stretches and range-of-motion exercises will prevent injuries.

As you can see, a thorough evaluation of physical fitness takes into account a variety of factors. What are your areas of strength and weakness? You may strengthen your overall fitness for a healthier, more active lifestyle by focusing on your areas of weakness.

5. Endurance Of The Cardiorespiratory

That's a lot, but it refers to your capacity to perform tasks like running, riding, or rapid walking without quickly becoming weary.

You may assess your heart rate, breathing rate, and endurance with a cardio fitness analysis provided by a trainer or fitness facility staff member.

Reasons You Should Get Fit

We all want to be in good shape. However, many people aspire to get in shape solely for appearance. However, there are many reasons to get in shape aside from appearance.

Getting in shape, in fact, can help with practically every aspect of self-improvement, from alleviating worry and low self-esteem to combating sleeplessness and aging.

While there's nothing wrong with wanting to get healthy so you can feel good about your appearance, working out solely for appearance isn't the ideal long-term incentive for working out and staying fit.

Though the word "exercise" has a single dictionary definition, our motivations for doing so are diverse - and extend far beyond the conventional goals of slimming down or toning up. Make no mistake about the best version of yourself. Exercising will help you get there, and the advantages are numerous.

Here are the top (10) reasons why you should get started right away;

1. Improves Overall Health

Getting in shape is akin to putting money aside for the future. If you want to live a long and healthy life, you must exercise! Fit people are always healthier than unfit people, even if they weigh more. So don't worry about how much you weigh. Just get healthy enough to maintain your health now and in the future.

2. Faster Metabolism

When you exercise, you burn calories both when you're moving and when you're not. Regular resistance exercise (such as weight-based workouts) will maximize your lean body mass while increasing your metabolic rate.

3. Reduces Stress, Anxiety And Depression

We've all heard that regular exercise improves your mood, but it does so much more.

Exercise releases neurotransmitters and endorphins that help with depression. You also get to boost your body temperature which has been known to reduce anxiety.

4. Improves Mental Performance And Work Productivity

We feel that exercise is essential for enhancing the overall quality of life particularly at work. Exercise not only boosts self-confidence in the job allowing you to take on leadership responsibilities and perform better but it also boosts general productivity and focuses.

5. Boosts Your Sexual Life

Your libido can be increased by regular exercise. Exercise
causes the brain to release endorphins which trigger the
production of sex hormones. These hormones calm the
body, lower blood pressure and cortisol levels, enhance
digestion, and lower heart rate.

6. Reduces Your Chances of Dementia

Several studies have showed that being active helps to
improve mental function and energy, lowering the risk of
dementia.

Physical activity can improve cognitive function in healthy
older people and may lower the likelihood of developing
cognitive impairment.

Dance courses, in particular, which involve learning abilities
such as memory and focus are very beneficial for people at
risk of *Alzheimer's disease*.

7. To Build Confidence

Seeing your genuine capabilities is the best way to increase
your confidence.

What does "becoming fit" entail? It could appear differently
to each person. One person's ability to perform 100 burpees
in a row is a significant feat that they could only achieve after

putting in a lot of effort to improve their strength and conditioning.

Even while someone else may have always believed it would be completely impossible for them to ever perform a handstand after months or even years of practice (this stuff takes time!), they are now beginning to feel as though they have perfected the talent.

Guess how these folks feel after accomplishing these goals? They not only became fitter, but their confidence also increased greatly.

8. Reduces Your Stress

Living in the current day is undeniably stressful, and it may be difficult to disconnect from work. How to manage stress via exercise is one of the difficulties we face. Clinical research have shown that those who have healthy lifestyles experience less stress and anxiety.

9. It Increases Your Fertility Rate

The gym is the place to go if you want a fruitful future filled with many offspring. Researchers from Harvard University have shown that men who exercise frequently have more sperm.

10.   Ensures Longevity

This is one of the most evident advantages of living a healthy lifestyle and is one of the causes for which most individuals look to engage in physical activity and consume a balanced diet.

There is proof that ties maintaining health with living longer which is good news for individuals who are motivated to get the most lifespan out of their body.

One research even estimated that quitting smoking, exercising frequently, and eating a nutritious diet, together with consuming alcohol sometimes might add up to 14 years to your life expectancy.

Simple Tips For Fitness Success

Numerous factors, like body mass index, waist size, body fat percentage, straight tests, and endurance exercises can be used to assess physical fitness.

The majority of individuals desire to reach their fitness objectives quickly and effectively. But becoming in shape is a process that demands a great deal of dedication and regularity.

Unfortunately, a lot of individuals stop exercising completely when the results aren't what they expected.

Despite the fact that getting in shape sounds like a tedious, time-consuming procedure, the benefits of making the effort to do so are numerous. So how can you maintain consistency in your exercise routine? Here are a few straightforward suggestions to help you succeed in your fitness goals.

➢ Keep Track Of Your Calories

Calories are a unit of energy that is commonly used to calculate the energy content of meals and drinks.

A dietary calorie is technically defined as the amount of energy necessary to raise the temperature of one kilogramme of water by one degree celsius.

Calories are used for fundamental tasks such as breathing and thinking, as well as daily activities like walking, talking, and eating.

Any extra calories you consume will be stored as fat and eating more than you burn will result in weight gain over time.

Keeping track of your daily calorie intake is the number one way to your fitness journey. Even though, it could be difficult to do but I will give you some tips on how to keep track of your calorie intake.

Best Way To Track calorie

A simple approach to tracking calories is to use an app or web tool to record your meals and track your food consumption.

Calorie counting is now reasonably simple to implement because of technological advancements.

10 Best Applications For Calorie Tracking

There are several applications and websites available to help ease the process by giving quick and easy ways to track the food you consume.

Even if you merely check your food consumption on an irregular basis, research suggests that those who do so lose more weight and keep it off longer.

The following are some of the most popular calorie-counting applications:

- MyFitness Pal

- Cronometer

- Lose it

- Lifesum

- MyNetDairy

- Calory

- Noom

- FatSecret

- SparkPeople

- MyPlate

NOTE: The majority of the calorie counting apps mentioned above are free. Although some have 'premium' alternatives while others are only a few pounds a month. Choose the one that works best for you and your monthly budget.

➢ Eat Healthy Low Calorie Food

Eating meals with a low calorie density is another approach to increase satisfaction while consuming fewer calories.

This applies to foods with a high water content, including several fruits and vegetables.

Studies repeatedly demonstrate that dieters who consume foods with a lower calorie density than those who consume foods with a higher calorie density lose more weight.

In one study, women who consumed soup, which has a low calorie density lost 50% more weight than those who consumed a snack high in calories.

Additionally, vegetables include a lot of soluble fibre, which has been linked to weight loss in some studies.The fact that soluble fibre is broken down by bacteria in the digestive tract is another advantage of it.

A byproduct of this process generates a fatty acid called *butyrate* which at least in rats is thought to have anti-obesity properties.

Simply put, you can lose weight by selecting meals with a low-calorie density such as high-fiber vegetables without reducing the amount of food you eat.

➢ Exercise Daily

Everyone has heard it a million times that regular exercise is good for you and can aid in weight loss and improves physically fitness. But if you're like many Americans, you're occupied, you work a desk job, and haven't changed your fitness routine yet. You can start whenever you choose which is a fantastic thing.

Adding more physical activity to your daily routine can be done gradually and subtly at first. Strive to exercise at the recommended rate for your age to get the most benefits. You will feel better, you'll be able to prevent or control many ailments and you might even live longer if you are successful.

Exercise and physical activity can improve your health and reduce your risk of developing diseases such as *type 2 diabetes, cancer, and cardiovascular disease*. Physical activity and exercise can provide both short-term and long-term health benefits.

Above all, regular physical activity can improve your overall quality of life. These advantages can be obtained with as little as 30 minutes of exercise per day.

Bottom Line: Working out at home broadens your possibilities for improving your daily exercise. It is more convenient and accessible than a gym. When trying to build a workout at home, your body weight is a fantastic place to start but if you want more, consider investing in multipurpose equipment. If scheduled workouts aren't your thing, try to incorporate natural movement into your day.

➢ Drink Water And Stay Hydrated

Just like our globe is composed of 71% water, our bodies are composed of about 60% water. As a result, besides oxygen, water is the most important thing for human survival on this planet. Given these realities, we must hydrate and restore our resources regularly.

Furthermore, hydration is essential when working out in the gym to get the most out of your body. Fluids are essential for keeping the body healthy. Water is necessary for sustaining a healthy heart, brain, and muscles, as well as for regulating our body temperature through sweat. *Staying hydrated throughout a workout enhances your general capacity to complete workouts, promotes sleep, aids in detoxification, and aids in weight loss.*

We frequently forget to hydrate properly during our workouts, which leads to dehydration. This can lead to serious issues such as muscle fatigue, excessive sweating due to an increase in our body temperatures and thus overheating and a problem with our mental functions which can lead to larger issues such as dizziness or fainting. We cannot emphasize enough how crucial it is to refill body fluids to avoid such complications.

➤ Take Multivitamin Supplements

The human body requires a wide and complex variety of vital nutrients to complete all of the tasks it has in a typical day. When one of these essential vitamins or minerals is deficient, the metabolic pathway that produces optimum efficiency breaks down and performance suffers. This is obviously NOT what you want!

Taking a high-potency multivitamin/multi-mineral formula may assist in ensuring the presence of those essential nutrients required for thousands of metabolic reactions.

Bodybuilders, athletes, and people who live an active lifestyle require more nutrients than the average person. So, if you think that grabbing the first one you see on the shelf will suffice, think again.

➢ Get Enough Good Sleep

There is a clear link between sleep quality and the amount and your immune system. You can maintain your immune system operating correctly by obtaining seven to eight hours of sleep every night.

When addressing health and weight, sleep and stress levels are frequently overlooked. Both are critical for the proper functioning of your body and hormones.

In fact, lack of sleep is one of the most significant risk factors for obesity. According to one study, short sleep duration increased the risk by 89 percent in children and 55 percent in adults.

Inadequate sleep can also increase hunger and cravings, resulting in a biological inclination for weight gain by affecting hunger hormones such as ghrelin and leptin.

Excessive stress can raise cortisol levels which are known to promote belly fat buildup and the risk of chronic western diseases such as type II diabetes and heart disease.

Making time for quality sleep and avoiding unneeded pressures in your life are therefore crucial.

How Low Calorie Helps In Getting Fit

Calorie counts and how low you should go are two of the most crucial diet concepts to comprehend. Never choose a diet that asks for less than 1,200 calories per day unless it is prescribed by a doctor. Never cut your daily calorie intake below 1,200, not because weight loss would happen too quickly, but because the opposite is frequently true.

Your metabolism will make every effort to hold onto the reserve energy it has saved as long as possible as a part of your basic survival. Naturally, fat is where that energy is stored. You will not be speeding your weight loss, you will be slowing it down and you will do so at the risk of other issues such as lower potassium or sugar levels.

These changes are the reason that some people pass out when they are on this type of starvation diet. You will also be lowering your resistance to illness and have such a low energy level, you will find it harder to get through the day.

Another point to consider when looking for *free diet plans is* to avoid those that suggest diet bars or shakes. You will not be physically satisfied since these usually digest too quickly. The other problem is you will not get enough fibre from them and they often contain ingredients you don't want like fructose com syrup which studies indicate hurts the metabolism.

How many calories should I consume daily?

Most of the time, when we consider calories, we consider how fatty food is. Again, calories are the quantity of energy that a food contains in terms of nutrition.

We will put on weight if we continually consume more energy than we require. We will begin to lose weight, fat, and eventually muscle mass if we consume insufficient energy.

The amount of energy required to raise the temperature of 1 gram (g) of water by 1°C is referred to as a calorie.

How many calories we consume depends on the kind and quantity of food we eat. The amount of calories in a food is frequently a decisive factor for dieters when selecting whether or not to consume it.

Given that the body consumes energy differently throughout the day, when and how we eat might also have an impact. Our level of activity, our body's energy-use efficiency, and our age all affect how much energy our bodies consume.

The ideal daily calorie intake is influenced by a variety of factors, including age, metabolism, level of physical activity, and others.

In general, women should consume 1,500–2,000 calories per day, whereas men should consume 2,500–3,000 calories every day.

Below is a chart of estimated daily calorie intake based on gender, age and activity level for individuals.

GENDER	AGE	SEDENTARY (CALORY)	ACTIVE (CALORY)
CHILD (BOY&GIRL)	2 - 3	1,000	1,000-1400
FEMALE	4 -8	1,200	1,400-1,600
	9 – 13	1,600	1,600-2,000
	14 – 18	1,800	2,000
	19 – 29	2,000	2,000-2,200
	30 – 49	1,800	2,000
	50+	1,600	1,800
MALE	4 -8	1,400	1,400-1,600
	9 – 13	1,800	1,800-2,200
	14 – 18	2,200	2,400-2,800
	19 – 29	2,400	2,600-2,800
	30 – 49	2,200	2,400-2,600
	50+	2,000	2,200-2,400

Low Calorie Breakfast Recipes

The beauty of breakfast is that you may jumpstart your day with a blast of taste and energy that sets your day off to a great start. But in reality, it's hard to find the time to have a nutritious breakfast that's beneficial since it's not everyone that has a tonne of time in the morning to commit to creating healthy morning meals while they're hurrying to go to work. That's where these healthy breakfast dishes come in though, as they will help you remain on track with your health objectives without spending a tonne of time. They're all easy to whip up, I guarantee!

➢ Cashew Butter & Rapsberry Smoothie

This smoothie blends tart fruit with creamy nut butter was created as an homage to the peanut butter and jelly sandwich. You may use this recipe's flexibility to swap out the *cashew butter for peanut or almond butter or the raspberries for strawberries or other fruit.*

Cashews are rich in monounsaturated fats and protein, both of which are good for the heart. In addition to adding a nice pink tint to your smoothie, frozen raspberries also provide it with 9 grams of fiber and 60% of the daily recommended amount of vitamin C.

Ingredients

- One tablespoon of cashew butter

- One cup of Pacific Foods Original Cashew Plant-Based Beverage

- ½ cup of cottage cheese

Procedure

- In a blender, combine all of the ingredients.

- Blend for 1 to 2 minutes on low, then 1 to 2 minutes on high or until smooth.

➢ Sweet Potato Banana Muffins

No matter the kind of diet someone follows, they can't resist these muffins. Furthermore, they have a delightful soft and moist texture with just a hint of sweetness. They are also devoid of gluten, dairy, and refined sugar. They are particularly enjoyable to indulge in throughout the winter because of the robust sweet potato taste and the scrumptious scented spices.

Make them into a healthy dessert that you may eat or prepare them for breakfast and enjoy with coffee or tea. *The sweet potatoes and bananas in this recipe are the sole sources of sweetness, yet you won't believe how filling these muffins are.*

Ingredients

- Two mashed bananas that are ripe

- 1 ¾ cups of almond flour

- ¼ cup of mashed sweet potato

- ¼ cup of tapioca flour

- Three raw eggs

- ¼ cup of unsweetened canned coconut cream

- One tablespoon of baking soda

- One tablespoon of baking powder

- One teaspoon of ginger powder

- One teaspoon of cinnamon powder

- ½ teaspoon of salt

Procedure

- Preheat the oven to 350°F.

- A 12-cup standard muffin tray should be lined with parchment paper or generously greased.

- Combine the bananas, eggs, sweet potato, and coconut cream in a medium bowl.

- Mix the almond flour, tapioca flour, baking powder, baking soda, cinnamon, ginger, and salt in a separate big basin.

- Just blend by gradually incorporating the wet components into the dry ones.

- The batter should be uniformly distributed throughout the muffin pan wells after preparation.

- Bake for 25 to 30 minutes.

- Remove from the oven and allow to cool before serving.

➢ Pancakes With Cashew Butter

This pancake recipe made with whole grains is enriched with a few foods that are excellent sources of nutrition for vegans. Each portion of this meal has 14 grammes of protein, making it the ideal breakfast for mornings when you need a little additional vigour.

Ingredients

- One cup of Buttermilk Flapjack & Waffle Mix by Kodiak Cakes

- One cup of the unsweetened hemp original beverage from Pacific Foods

- One tablespoon of cashew butter

- 50g of blueberries

- Half a cup of strawberries

- Two tablespoons of honey

Procedure

- In a medium bowl, combine the hemp beverage with the pancake mix and whisk until smooth.

- Pour ½ cup of pancake mix into a cast-iron skillet that has been well-seasoned and heat over medium-high heat.

- After approximately 3 minutes, when the pancake begins to bubble, flip it over and cook it for an additional minute.

- Each pancake should have a spoonful of nut butter on top before being stacked.

- Place berries on top of the stack and sprinkle honey over them.

- Breakfast is ready!

➢ Pear Cardamom Oat Smoothie

Bartlett pears are excellent for smoothies. This is because, when mature, they become juicy and tender. They are a wonderful source of vitamin C and a great source of fibre.

Whether you add oats straight to the smoothie or use a plant-based oat beverage, oats offer a creamy and sweet smoothie base. The oat beverage from Pacific Foods is a fantastic source of calcium that is lactose and soy-free and also has vitamin D. And it contains organic oats, which naturally sweeten it! An oat beverage is ideal for a dish that nods to a pear crisp in flavour because it often works well in baked products.

Ingredients

- ¼ cup of organic Bob's Red Mill Organic Old Fashioned Rolled Oats

- One cup of Pacific Foods Original Plant-Based Beverage with Oats

- ½ Bartlett pear

- Two teaspoons of honey (wildflower or clover)

- ½ cup of ice

- ¼ teaspoon of ground cardamom

Procedure

- In a blender, combine all of the ingredients.

- Blend on low for 1 to 2 minutes, then on high for 1 to 2 minutes or until smooth.

➢ **Black Bean Omelet**

Which would you prefer: a spinach omelet from a restaurant with roughly 1,000 calories, or a 330-calorie omelet with an oozing middle of black beans and cheese?

Ingredients

- ¼ teaspoon of cumin

- Spicy sauce

- Eight raw eggs

- Salt and black pepper

- Half cup of feta cheese

- Pico de Gallo or store-bought salsa

- Avocado slices (optional)

Procedure

- In a food processor, pulse the black beans with the lime juice, cumin, and a few dashes of hot sauce until the mixture resembles refried beans. If required, add a little water to assist.

- Heat a small nonstick pan over medium heat after coating it with nonstick cooking spray, some butter, or olive oil.

- Two eggs should be cracked into a bowl and beat with some salt and pepper.

- The eggs should be added to the pan, stirred with a spatula, and then the cooked egg on the bottom is lifted to make room for the raw egg to slip below.

- Spoon two tablespoons of feta cheese and a quarter of the black bean mixture down the centre of the omelet when it is almost completely set.

- Utilizing the spatula, fold over a third of the egg to cover the centre mixture. Carefully slide the omelet onto a dish, flipping it over with the spatula just before doing so to create a single, fully folded omelet.

- To create four omelets, repeat the process with the remaining ingredients.

- Avocado slices, pico de gallo, and a little additional feta crumbles can be used as garnish.

Nutrition: 330cal

➤ Pastrami And Swiss Egg Sandwich (325 cal)

It's the ideal breakfast sandwich you've been looking for, and it's loaded with protein and fiber.

Ingredients

- Half tablespoon of butter

- Cut into strips, 4 oz. lean pastrami (or turkey pastrami)

- Six raw eggs

- Two tablespoons of milk

- Black pepper and salt

- Four low-fat slices of Swiss cheese

- Four English muffins made with whole wheat, gently toasted

Procedure

- Over medium heat, melt the butter in a large nonstick pan.

- Pastrami should be added and sautéed for 2 to 3 minutes.

- Reduce the heat to a low setting.

- In a bowl, crack all the six eggs and add salt & pepper to taste, along with the milk.

- Whisk the mixture together and add to the pan after whisking.

- Stir often with a wooden spoon.

- Scrape the bottom as they set.

- On the bottom of each English muffin, put a slice of Swiss cheese.

- While serving, divide the scrambled eggs among the muffins and top with the muffin tops.

Nutrition: 325cal

➤ Banana Pancakes

Two things happen when yoghurt and cottage cheese are used in these pancakes: It increases the amount of protein served at breakfast and aids in creating the lightest, moistest pancakes you've ever had. Fresh banana slices may always be added to the batter, and as they touch the skillet, they caramelize into golden-brown discs of sweetness. However, the real key to this recipe is the batter, which should now be your go-to pancake base.

Ingredients

- One cup of plain Greek yoghurt

- One cup of ricotta or cottage cheese that is low in fat

- Three raw eggs

- One lemon juice

- One cup of White whole wheat flour

- ½ teaspoon of baking soda

- A dash of salt

- Two sliced bananas

- Warm maple syrup

Procedure

- Yoghurt, cottage cheese, eggs, and lemon juice should all be combined in a bowl and must be whisked thoroughly.

- In another basin, combine the salt, baking soda, and flour.

- Stir just until combined before adding the flour mixture to the yoghurt mixture.

- Melt the butter in a frying pan over low heat.

- After sprinkling the pan with nonstick cooking spray, add two spoonfuls of the batter.

- Add three to four banana slices to each pancake as soon as the batter touches the pan, gently pushing them into the batter.

- Cook until the tops start to boil for three to five minutes.

- The second side of the pancakes should be cooked for a further two minutes or until golden brown.

- If desired, top the pancakes with more banana slices after adding some syrup.

Nutrition : 320cal

➢ Spinach And Ham Quiche

The quiche is the perfect culinary chameleon because it can be cooked with a wide variety of flavour combinations and because it tastes just as wonderful for supper with a glass of red wine as it does for breakfast with a cup of coffee. Or divide the difference: This quiche recipe is perfect for meal prep since it can be made on Sunday night for supper and then you can bring a slice to work on Monday.

Ingredients

- One frozen pie shell, thawed and fork-pricked

- ½ tablespoon of olive oil

- One minced garlic clove

- ½ bunch cleaned, dried, and stemmed spinach

- Two oz smoked ham cut into ¼ inch cubes

- ½ cup of shredded Swiss cheese

- Four raw eggs

- One cup of milk

- ¼ cup of half-and-half

- ½ teaspoon of salt

- Pinch of nutmeg

Procedure

- Once the oven is preheated, the pie shell should be baked for about 10 minutes, or until lightly toasted but not browned.

- Olive oil should be heated in a large skillet or pot over medium heat while the oven heats up and the shell bakes.

- After 30 seconds of heating the oil, the spinach should be added.

- The spinach should be cooked for 5 minutes or until totally wilted.

- Squeeze the spinach firmly to remove any excess water before adding it, and then combine with the ham, cheese, eggs, milk, half-and-half, and spinach in a large mixing dish.

- Add nutmeg and salt for seasoning.

- Fill the warm pastry shell with the egg mixture.

- Bake the quiche for 12 minutes or until the top is gently browned.

Nutrition: 260cal

➢ Fruit And Granola Yoghurt Parfait

Fruit-flavored yoghurts are essentially ice cream that has been elevated. Any fruit-on-the-bottom brand's label will demonstrate what we mean. High-fructose corn syrup probably appears on the ingredients list far earlier than genuine fruit. Therefore, it is always preferable to get plain Greek yoghurt that is high in protein and probiotics and to add the actual fruit yourself.

In this recipe, we layer it for aesthetic purposes and add granola for crunch. This delectable parfait is rich enough to pass for dessert, but it also has a combination of protein and fiber, which is precisely what you need to start the day or as a snack.

Ingredients

- One cup of strawberry slices (any juicy fruit will work well here if you want to sub in things like raspberries, blackberries, kiwi, and mangoes).

- A half-cup of blueberries

- Two teaspoons of sugar

- Four thinly cut mint leaves

- One container of plain low-fat Greek yoghurt (8 oz)

- ¼ cup of granola

Procedure

- In a bowl, combine the fruit, sugar, and mint. Let stand for three to four minutes.

- Place half of the yoghurt, half of the fruit, and half of the granola in a bowl or glass. Repeat with the remaining yoghurt, fruit, and granola.

- Any remaining fruit juice should be poured on top.

Nutrition: 330cal

➤ Banana Nutella Crepes (260 cal)

There isn't anything that doesn't go well with Nutella. Crepes appear to have been made just to house fresh banana slices and hazelnut-chocolate, at least that's what you'll be thinking as you knife and fork your way through one of these simple but oh-so-decadent sweet delights.

The reality is that all types of dessert crepes are delicious but nothing beats this combo. Even though Nutella, the Italian chocolate-hazelnut spread you may already be obsessed with is more of a European treat, standard chocolate sauce will elicit fits of uncontrollable pleasure in the United States.

Ingredients

Crepes butter component

- ¼ cup of Nutella

- Two cut and peeled bananas

- Sugar used for confections (optional)

Regarding the crepe batter

- ½ cup of flour

- One big raw egg

- One tablespoon of melted butter

- Pinch of salt

- Six tablespoon of low-fat milk

- 1/8 cup of water

Procedure

- Nonstick pan should be heated to medium heat.

- Coat the pan with enough butter.

- Add 2 tablespoons of the crepe batter and swish the pan (use a rubber spatula to help, if needed).

- For the bottom to turn a deep golden brown, cook the first side for 3 to 4 minutes.

- Once the crepe is flipped over, spread a tablespoon of Nutella down the center and top with a few slices of banana.

- The bottom should be golden brown after cooking for an additional 3 to 4 minutes.

- As soon as the filling is tucked inside the crepe, fold the sides over it.

- Slices of banana and confectioners sugar can be added as garnishes if desired.

- To make three additional crepes, repeat.

Nutrition: 330cal

Low Calorie Lunch Ideas

Take a look at these delectable, convenient boxed lunch meals under **300 calories** to keep you content and full!

- ## Healthy Chicken Lettuce Wraps

  These chicken wraps with Asian influences are the ideal taco substitute.

  Despite how much we all adore tacos, there is no getting around the extra calories in the tortillas. With these, you can enjoy delicious finger foods with half the calories!

  Instead, use lettuce for a great crunchy texture and to keep things light.

- ## Shrimp Tacos With Cilantro Lime Sauce

  Using corn tortillas is the key to keeping your tacos free of carbohydrates, and the beautiful thing about tacos is that they taste amazing with only a few simple toppings.

  Only a few simple items are required to make these flavorful shrimp tacos. I recommend trying a bag of store-bought broccoli slaw. It usually contains shredded vegetables and gives your cuisine a wonderful colour.

  Plus, it adds a lovely crunch to your soft shrimp!

➢ Steak Salad

You can still enjoy a delicious steak even though you're seeking something lower in calories.

The ingredients called for in this recipe are: salt, pepper, paprika, garlic powder, onion powder, and dried thyme.

- All the ingredients should be added to cubed steak before it is fried. But I believe there's a simpler approach!

- Prepare a steak according to standard procedure.

- Get your pan sizzling hot, then cook the food for a few minutes on each side before letting it rest.

- Cut the food through, then serve it in strips.

- By doing so, you reduce the possibility of overcooking and drying out your meat.

➢ Jambalaya With Shrimps And Sausage

Jambalaya is an excellent recipe to prepare when you wish to reduce your calorie intake. *It's full of vegetables, herbs, and spices and is naturally low in carbs.*

Because it's already quite nutritious, you'll only need to make a few changes to keep it under 300 calories per serving.

The simplest change is to replace the Andouille sausage with something leaner.

To make it even lower, replace the rice with cauliflower rice!

➢ Skinny Potato Pancake

Potatoes are a common ingredient in most homes because they're tasty, adaptable, and inexpensive.

Giving them up is difficult, which is why this low-calorie potato side dish is ideal when attempting to reduce calorie intake.

Since you're using mashed potatoes, all you have to do is cook them in the pan until they get a lovely golden crust.

➢ Skinny Burrito Bowls

Burrito bowls are free of carbohydrates and healthier.

The nice thing about burritos is that you can easily replace the rice in them with quinoa or cauliflower rice, and the food will still taste just like a burrito.

Although ground turkey is a terrific low-calorie alternative, I personally prefer mine with shredded chicken.

➢ Shrimp And Asparagus Stir Fry

Asparagus has a wonderful crunch even after being cooked and that is what I enjoy about it the most.

The shrimp can also really stand out because the flavour isn't overbearing. Furthermore, since neither the shrimp nor the vegetables require much cooking time in the pan, *this two-ingredient stir fry may be quickly put together.*

➢ Healthy Tortilla Pizza

This might be a nice compromise for when you're craving pizza with a thin crust and small toppings. However, if you prefer a thick pizza crust and lots of toppings, this isn't the best choice for you as this isn't as healthy as a pizza with thin crust.

Brown rice flour tortillas taste delicious and are a great low-carb alternative. It's time to try brown rice flour tortillas if you've never done so.

➢ Teriyaki Chicken

Although it may not seem like a meal that can be made in about 15 minutes, I assure you that it is actually pretty simple!

- Water, soy sauce, honey, brown sugar, rice vinegar, sesame oil, garlic, ginger, and cornstarch should all be combined in a small pot. Stir everything together until it seems smooth.

- Simply pour it over the chicken and allow the heat from the pan to thicken it.

- Serve and enjoy!

The benefit of making your own is that you have complete control over the ingredients.

Feel free to switch to coconut sugar or fully cut out sugar from your diet!

➢ Chicken Fried Rice

One of the most delicious options for the holiday lunch menu is chicken fried rice. This dish is incredibly simple to prepare and has a tonne of chicken, veggies, and spices.

This delicious lunch made with eggs, cooked rice, chicken, carrots, green onions, garlic, frozen peas, and other kitchen essentials will be enjoyed by all.

You could also use leftover chicken to prepare this lunch.

➢ Ground Turkey Sweet Potato Skillet

The sweet potato flavours complement the turkey well, making this a delicious lunch option.

Because it contains sweet potatoes, ground turkey, and a variety of spices, this meal is extremely nutritious.

You'll probably have some leftovers to snack on during the week because this is a large skillet meal.

Low Calorie Dinner Ideas

When trying to eat healthily, *salads are a popular healthy meal option, especially around dinnertime*. They are full-packed with healthy vegetables.

On the other side, eating salads five times a week could become monotonous, especially if you use the same mix. This might cause you to get tired of your usual meal and choose something wholly unhealthy in its place.

These under 300-calorie dinner dishes for weight loss are a fun way to mix things.

➢ Vegan Taco Salad

Vegan taco salad is a cost-effective, healthful, vegan, and gluten-free way to prepare meals. Try making taco salad at home if you're searching for an easy and quick plant-based meal.

Black bean, corns, mixed greens, tomatoes, avocado, crispy tortilla strips, and salad cream are the only easy items you'll need for this 10-minute salad. This meal is one of my favourite under-300-calorie dinners that is also beneficial to our health.

➢ Thai Peanut Chicken Salad

The healthiest option for a quick meal that provides nutrients and vitamins is salad. Try making Thai peanut chicken salad dish if you enjoy salads. There is a lot of chicken, peanuts, veggies, and peanut dressing in it.

It's a straightforward meal that takes about 20 minutes to prepare. Peanut-lime-ginger dressing, tender chicken, crunchy cabbage or coleslaw, red bell peppers, scallions, and chopped peanuts make this fresh, healthful, straightforward, and ideal lunch.

➢ Tuna Salad

Tuna salad is a nutritious and protein-rich dish suitable for all ages.

It is tasty, easy, and quick creamy texture bursting with flavour. It goes great with lettuce wraps, keto bread, or your favourite keto crackers or cheese crisps!

➢ Stir Fry Zucchini Noodles

When you crave noodles but need a healthy supper, the finest option for getting a nutritious and delectable meal for dinner (or sometimes for lunch) is stir-fried zucchini noodles.

Making these noodles at home simply takes 30 minutes and is loaded with vegetables.

This low-carb variation helps you stick to your diet and stay healthy. In addition, you can include any vegetables, poultry, or other ingredients.

➤ Skinny Oven Fried Chicken

Thin oven-fried chicken dish should be your best buddy if you're short on time and need a dinner you can make quickly and with little supervision.

Making your own with cornflakes and breadcrumbs can help the chicken get even more crispy.

The recipe's simplicity makes it the best feature.

All you have to do is watch for the chicken to turn golden brown after seasoning it and placing it in the oven.

To have leftover chicken for a salad later in the week, you may also put a lot of chicken on a sheet pan before cooking it.

➤ Steak Salad

You'll probably wind up making this low-calorie dinner recipe on a regular basis because it's so wonderful.

A top-notch steak, some leafy greens, and a delectable dressing are the ingredients you need.

Whatever suits your unique taste, you can add a wide variety of dressings that will perfectly complement the steak.

To step up this recipe, you may add whatever other ingredients you desire, such as roasted cherry tomatoes, onions, or crumbled blue cheese.

➢ Shrimp Stir Fry

If you don't use the high-calorie oil, shrimp stir fry is nutritious. It is also easy to make and not time-consuming.

It contains all the same fantastic vegetables and seasonings as any other stir fry. It can be made quickly and is ideal for those times when you're unsure of what to serve for dinner.

➢ Healthy Minestrone Soup

A traditional healthy soup like minestrone can be filling without being overly heavy.

To make this variation of minestrone soup as tasty as possible, fresh vegetables including zucchini noodles, butternut squash, and greens are used.

Despite being sweet, minestrone includes a tomato-based broth, making it one of the meals with fewer than 300 calories.

Try it with some quinoa instead of adding noodles, which might increase the calorie count.

Additionally, you won't feel bloated after eating it if quinoa is used.

➢ Lemon Chickpea Salad

Chickpeas are nutritious food that are abundant in protein and vitamins. They also make you healthier. Lemon chicken salad is the perfect option if you're looking for a quick, high-protein dinner.

With lemon, cilantro, and other ingredients, this salad can be prepared in just 10 minutes and is vegan. You need to try this meal.

➢ Baked Tilapia With Lemon Capers

Baking Tilapia is a breeze, and a lemon-caper sauce transforms it into a delectable entrée.

The lemon sauce provides citrus flavours, and when combined with the salty capers, you'll have a bright and light supper that's ideal for hot days when you need something refreshing.

The best aspect about this dish is how simple it is to make.

- Simply combine the capers, lemon juice, salt, and pepper in a small bowl and spread it over the tilapia fillet.

- Toss everything in the oven and wait for perfection to emerge.

You'll love this flavour profile because it's likely to be a nice change from your normal meals.

Tips To Succeed With Calorie Counting

- **Be ready**: Get a calorie counter app or online tool, choose how you'll measure or estimate quantities, and create a meal plan before you begin.

- **Observe food labels**: Calorie counting is made much easier by the wealth of information on food labels. Make sure you review the suggested serving amount listed on the packaging.

- **Eliminate temptation:** Eliminate junk food. You'll be able to pick healthier snacks as a result, which will make reaching your goals simpler.

- **Try to lose weight gradually and steadily**: Avoid calorie restriction that is too extreme. Even though you'll lose weight more quickly, you could feel unwell and be less likely to follow your plan.

- **Fuel your workouts**: *The most effective weight loss plans include nutrition and exercise*. Eat enough food so that you can have the energy to work out.

Best Exercises To Lose Weight At Home

Your overall health depends on exercise. Weight loss and good health are associated. A person is more susceptible to conditions including hypertension, diabetes, cholesterol, and other cardiovascular issues if they have a higher body mass index. In order to effectively manage chronic illnesses, exercise becomes absolutely essential.

In addition to aiding in weight loss and fitness, exercise offers many other advantages. You feel happier after working out, and it also strengthens your bones and lowers your risk of developing numerous chronic conditions.

People sometimes stop exercising because they don't have the time to go to the gym or because they can't afford to hire a personal trainer to help them on their fitness path.

In order to help you get stronger, fitter, and healthier, I'd like to offer the **top five** fitness regimens that you may do at home.

a. Aerobics Exercises

One of the best workouts for losing weight is walking. A terrific workout for burning calories is brisk walking. It is a workout regimen that can fit into your daily activities and has little impact on your joints.

Running and jogging are regarded as the best workouts for losing weight. These workouts include the entire body and are integrated. Your legs will get stronger, and it works wonders on tummy fat.

The pace is the main distinction between jogging and running. Running will be at about 10 kph, while jogging is between 6 and 9 kph.

Exercise Routine

- Start by engaging in 15 minutes of walking exercise.

- For the subsequent 15 minutes, pick up the tempo and begin jogging.

- Run for another 15 minutes, picking up the pace each minute.

- After 10 minutes, pick up the pace once more and resume jogging.

- Walk for five minutes while letting your body relax and slowing your speed.

Bottom Line

The combination of these three exercises (walking, running and jogging) will undoubtedly help you maintain a healthy and appropriate body weight and increase your muscular strength.

Running and jogging will help you burn about 375 calories every 30 minutes of activity and 300 calories per 30 minutes of activity respectively.

b. Squats

Squats are muscle-strengthening workouts. The major goal of this workout is to strengthen the lower body. Squats assist to burn calories and keep fat from building in your lower body. This workout improves your mobility and balance. To get better results, a beginner should aim for three sets of 12-15 reps of at least one form of squat.

Exercise Routine

- Stand erect with your feet wider than your hips apart and your toes pointing forward.

- Push your hips back by bending your ankles and knees.

- Keep your heels and toes firmly planted on the ground as you crouch.

- Pose yourself parallel to the floor with your knees bent at a 90-degree angle.

- Return to standing by pushing your heels together to straighten your legs.

This activity burns between 19 - 44 calories every 5 minutes (100 - 222 calories every 25 minutes).

c. Skipping/Jumping Rope

Skipping exercise gives your entire body a workout, boosts your metabolism, and helps you burn calories quickly.

Regular exercise will calm you down and aid with sadness and anxiety. This exercise also raises your heart rate, which causes your blood to move through your body more quickly and keeps your heart in better and healthier shape. This activity maintains the health and function of your lungs and heart.

Exercise Routine

- Stand with your back straight on a level surface.
- Make sure your feet are planted firmly and facing forward.
- Keep your hand close to your thighs, straight and facing downward.
- Leap off the ground, allowing your rope to pass below you as you pull it back.
- Repeat these actions while steadily quickening your jumps.

Bottom Line: Everybody has a unique body which causes the procedure to produce different results. Skipping will undoubtedly assist you in burning more calories than you consume, which is the only way to lose weight.

This type of activity burns around 1300 calories each hour.

d. Plank

One of the most efficient total-body exercises is the plank pose. The fact that Plank addresses the majority of the body's major muscle groups is its greatest benefit. *Your hips, back, shoulders, arms, chest, and core muscles are all strengthened as a result.* Along with these advantages, plank workouts assist in swiftly burning extra body fat and calories.

It is an exercise that sounds straightforward and easy but is highly demanding and severe. The plank exercise is an excellent illustration of how your results will improve as you work out longer. For quicker and more effective results, concentrate on maintaining the plank posture for a longer time.

There are several plank variants that focus on various body parts and muscle groups. Each variant is incredibly beneficial and maintains your posture, body balance, endurance, and core strength growing. These variation are:

- The Extended Arm Plank

The Extended Arms Plank is another name for the *Standard Plank*. The candidates for this role are newcomers who want to strengthen their core. This exercise is excellent for enhancing digestion and metabolic function. The extended arms plank variation is also the same as the *forearm plank variation. This exercise focuses on the core, arms, shoulders, and back.*

Exercise Routine

- Your hands should be level on the floor, your elbows should be tucked under your shoulders, and your core should be tight.

- Raise yourself slowly until your body is in a straight line from your knees to your head while maintaining your forearms and knees on the ground.

- Maintain the posture for as long as you can.

- ## The Reverse Plank

The Reverse Plank is a variant of the conventional plank that is executed backward. *You can stretch your body very well with this exercise.* It is a physical activity that helps your body burn off excess calories and fat. *Your gluteal, back, chest, shoulders, and core muscles are all strengthened as a result of this exercise.*

Exercise Routine

- Sit down and place your legs out in front of you.

- Put your hands behind your hips to support your upper body.

- To elevate your hips, straighten your hand, and align your body in a straight line.

- Keep holding this posture for 50-60 seconds.

- 20 to 30 times each should be used for these processes and techniques.

- **The Mountain Climbers**

This vigorous plank exercise variant is regarded as one of the best. It is a total-body exercise that helps the body burn off extra calories and fat. *The biceps, hamstrings, core, triceps, and chest are the muscles that this exercise specifically targets.*

Exercise Routine

- Take a push-up or a standard plank position.

- Right now, bend your right knee and bring it up to your chest.

- Return your right knee to its original position by pushing it.

- Now flex your left knee such that it is close to your chest.

- Bring your left knee back to its starting position.

- Repeat the previous processes for 20-25 times.

e. Yoga

Yoga, *a 5000-year-old practice*, has been shown to be an excellent weight loss therapy. It is thought to have been created by Rishis and Brahmans and consists of five essential principles.

The principles are:

> ➢ Exercise
>
> ➢ Diet
>
> ➢ Breathing
>
> ➢ Relaxation
>
> ➢ Meditation

Yoga and healthy nutrition work well together to help you lose weight while also keeping your body physically fit and mind healthy. It also promotes consciousness and your relationship with your body.

Yoga for diabetes can also help you decrease your blood sugar levels.

Yoga poses are essential aspect of weight loss. Yoga positions primarily aim to improve concentration and muscle tone. To reap the most advantages from yoga, your body should become used to certain positions.

Yoga positions that should be practiced for weight loss include:

> ➢ Shoulder Pose

> ➢ Triangle Pose

> ➢ Bridge Pose

> ➢ Plank Pose

> ➢ Bow Pose

I highly recommend you watch a detailed video on YouTube to know how to do all these poses.

- To do that, just search for "How to shoulder pose/stand" on YouTube and watch any video of your choice among the videos YouTube recommends for you.

- Repeat the process to watch all the videos on all poses.

This type of activity burns between 180 and 460 calories per session (highly dependent on the type, intensity, and duration of the session).

NOTE: The number of calories burnt indicated above are only estimates. The actual quantity will vary depending on a variety of factors such as your *weight, age, fitness level, the intensity of your activity, and the length of time you devote to each exercise.*

The Best Time To Exercise

The optimal time to complete your regular workout programme is probably early in the morning. The primary reason for this is that *exercising on an empty stomach is the most effective approach to burn stored fat*.

Even though the early alarm clocks anger you at first, they will gradually become a positive habit for you. Assume you get up every morning at 7 a.m. This causes your biological clock to shift early, causing you to become fatigued quicker in the evening or at night. This assists in sticking to the timetable.

How much water should you drink in a day?

A normal human body requires roughly *two litres* of water every day for optimum metabolism. *Drinking adequate water has health advantages such as reducing constipation, keeping good skin, and avoiding acne.* However, consuming more water than the body requires might lead to water intoxication.

Having said that, the usual norm for water consumption is eight - ounce glasses per day. Any suggested dosage, however, must be modified for a variety of circumstances, including health conditions and dietary requirements.

The following recommendations for a healthy total water intake are provided by the European Food Safety Authority (EFSA).

Group	Recommended Water Intake (Liters)
Infants 0 – 6 months 6 – 12 months	 100 – 190 ML (From Breast Milk) 0.8 – 1.0L

Children	
1 -2 years	1.2L
3 – 4 years	1.4L
5 – 8 years	1.6L
9 – 14 years (F)	1.9L
9 – 14 years (M)	2.1L
15 – 19 years (F)	2.5L
15 – 19 years (M)	3.0L
Adult	
Women	2.7L
Men	3.7L

Vitamins That Increase Muscle Mass And Fitness

Anyone embarking on a fitness program hopes to gain muscle mass and become more fit. Not only is fitness beneficial to cardiovascular health, but it also aids with weight loss. Unfortunately, a poor diet and inadequate supplementation can undo most of the effort. Muscle health is dependent on vitamins and minerals.

Make sure that these vitamins in particular are included in any fitness goals.

- **Vitamin C**

    A *Vitamin C* pill taken before or after exercise can improve performance significantly. *Vitamin C* is essential for cell and tissue formation. That means people should notice an increase in muscular growth.

    And as we get older, *Vitamin C* may become even more important for muscle growth. When taking a *Vitamin C* supplement, people over 50, particularly men, retain more muscle mass.

- **Vitamin B12**

    Vitamin B12 is involved in hundreds of minor but critical bodily activities. The water-soluble *Vitamin B12* aids in the formation of DNA, nerve cells, blood cells, and other tissues.

The vitamin can aid in a variety of ways. First, the supplement aids in energy generation, which can aid in general fitness.

Vitamin B12 also aids in the metabolization of protein, which is directly absorbed by the muscles. Getting enough Vitamin *B12* can help anyone achieve their fitness objectives.

- **Vitamin D**

  The body creates *Vitamin D* in reaction to sun exposure, earning it the nickname "the sunshine vitamin." Numerous processes, including the absorption of minerals like calcium, phosphorus, maintaining bone and brain health, depend on *Vitamin D*.

  Unexpectedly, *Vitamin D* can work wonders for the growth of muscles. According to research, those with high *Vitamin D* levels had more lean muscle mass.

  Additionally, the applicants in these investigations displayed superior muscle performance.

  For a daily supply, 20 to 30 minutes of direct sunlight is required. If you can't do that, consider taking a *Vitamin D* supplement.

- **Biotin (B Complex)**

  One of the B complex vitamins and a necessary component for numerous bodily processes is *biotin*. Popular uses of the vitamin include hair and skin.

  In contrast, *biotin's* main job is to turn food into energy, which might improve fitness levels. Furthermore, the increased protein production will be advantageous to muscles.

  Although it can be obtained as a supplement, biotin can be found in meat, eggs, nuts, and some dairy products.

Conclusion

Anyone may begin a fitness program that is suited to their own requirements. Success requires being consistent. You can't expect to get your dream six-pack or become an elite athlete over night. To adapt to new demands, such as breaking old habits, your body requires time.

In order to make your fitness journey a part of you, design a timetable or get a daily planner to write down your daily activities and include all the above *tips for fitness success* in it as this will help you track your fitness journey.

Be Consistent And Persistent

Consistency will first aid in your goal-achieving. For this, frequent exercise is necessary. Let's say you decide to work out three times per week, try to stick to this consistency. Your plans will occasionally be derailed by life. It occurs! You will succeed, though, provided you continue to practice excellent behavior and exercise frequently.

Secondly, maintaining focus requires a great deal of persistence. There will be times when your exercise program reaches a particularly challenging point or shows no improvement. This is normal! You will succeed if you don't veer off track.

Measure Your Progress

Finally, you must constantly assess your development! Why is this crucial? How can you tell whether you are really progressing significantly toward your fitness objectives? You won't be able to tell if you've improved until you record your achievements and progress on paper. This might relate to your weight fluctuation, blood pressure, mile time, bench press repetition count, and much more. *Always keep a progress journal!*

About The Author

Lateefah Raji is an author, a graphic designer, a digital content creator, a programmer and a profitability coach. She enjoys giving everything she knows back to the society.

She can be reached for consultation via;

Email: lateefahraj@gmail.com

Twitter: lateefahraj

Instagram: lateefahraj